Hypothalamusly Speaking
Uncle Sug

Contents

Dedication

Acknowledgments

Disclaimer

Introduction

Chapter 1
Why Me

Chapter 2
30–60 Day Release

Dedication
Rip
Marilyn marlene booker

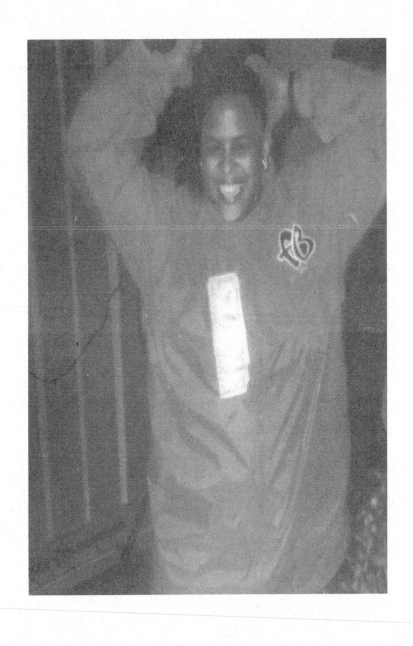

This book is a perfect example of a positive manifestation from a negative situation. I had no direction in my life until after my sister's passing. Her death taught me to seek only the positive no matter the circumstance; to only focus on what I can control. As long as I am alive, to remain thankful. Always have an attitude of gratitude. Grieve, and let go! Always strive to be better than I am today. Never be satisfied, but always be happy. Be different. She is the reason for all of my improvements. Marlene is responsible for every accomplishment I will achieve in the future. She is the reason I read books every day. I love and miss you more than words can express.

Thanks, SIS!

You should thank her too!

Acknowledgments

My sincere gratitude is extended

to all the special people who allowed me hours of their time to interview them and answer so many personal questions I asked.

Extra special thanks to the hundreds, or maybe even thousands, of doctors, whistleblowers, and courageous authors who exposed these corporations and their tactics.

And to all the references listed at the end of this book, thanks for providing the world with information and products to assist the human race in having vibrant and superb health.

Disclaimer

Many consider this to be an excellent work of fiction, yet inspired by true stories. I am not a medical doctor. I am not writing this to diagnose, cure, or treat any disease. I have no medical training.

I'm an investigating reporter/ journalist exercising my rights as such.

I do not sell any products.

I do not promote any products.

I have no financial interest in any company that sells

products.

I am not paid in any way on the sale of any product.
As a journalist, I am writing this manuscript based on real life experiences and observations for entertainment purposes.

I am not offering any medical advice.

If you choose to do anything in this book, you and only you are fully responsible!

If you have a disease or any medical problem, please, for your own safety, consult with a licensed health care provider and/or your doctor.

Some names, locations, dates, and events may have been modified or fictionalized, but were generated from reality.

This disclaimer has to be added due to the litigious nature of today's world and anticipated attacks, criticisms, and attempts to suppress and discredit this information.

Introduction

IF IT'S EVER REPORTED THAT GEORGE E. BOOKER II WAS FOUND DEAD BECAUSE OF A DRUG OVERDOSE OR SUICIDE, PLEASE DON'T BELIEVE IT! I CAN PROMISE

YOU IT WAS A MURDER!

I want you to understand that these are not my ideas.

The information being presented to you are proven methods from sources all around the world.

I am not a doctor. I have no medical training. I am not offering any medical advice.

I'm just a concerned reporter/ journalist/consumer advocate/ rapper/producer and US citizen presenting information that has been presented to me.

While working as an intern for WTAM 1100, The Mike Trivisonno Show (much love,

Triv), I had the pleasure of associating with, meeting, and interviewing current and former NFL and NBA coaches, players, general managers, TV show hosts, musicians, news and sports broadcasters, radio hosts, comedians, entertainers, doctors, personal trainers, college professors, congressmen, and authors.

I've read hundreds of books and articles and watched multiple documentaries and films about food, drugs, disease, and obesity.

The information I began to learn became shockingly scary.

The epidemic of obesity and

illness in our world today has become more of a problem than ever before.

Being overweight can lead to so many other problems physically and mentally.

One Sunday, after a lovely Mass at St. Agnes Our Lady of Fatima, some friends and I went shopping at Whole Foods, and somehow, we were discussing obesity. One of my sources gave me a five-question survey to ask five people who were overweight. My source also told me the answers each person would give.

My source then went on to say, "Ask as many people as you

want; that's just a small test to open your eyes." Here are the five questions and answers.

- Do you eat any fast food or restaurant food? (yes)
- Do you use 100 percent organic cooking oils only? (no)

- Do you eat fresh, organic fruits and vegetables only? (no)

- Do you eat a large, 100 percent organic breakfast every morning? (no)

- Do you do internal

cleansing regularly? (no)

My source made it clear to me that the questions and answers are not about what the overweight individual is doing now, but what was being done all the years leading up to their current condition.

So I immediately started as soon as we parted ways and asked the first person (I will not name names for obvious reasons; LOL). And wow, what do you know, a perfect five for five.

Me being the skeptic I am, thought to myself, "Yeah, OK,

that's just the first one; let's see about the next person."

Not only did this person go five for five, the next eight people went five for five!

That's when it all started for me, the idea to interview one hundred overweight people. After I got all the information I needed from them, I decide I would interview one hundred more people who successfully released thirty pounds or more.

The results were mind blowing! I can't explain how I was feeling hearing these real life stories from these people.

Imagine being face to face with

a woman who released 216 pounds in less than 120 days!

At the time I made the decision to interview people, I had no intention of writing a book.

I was doing this for my own personal education.

This book was encouraged by people I know telling me to write it.

So here it is. The world's most powerful information on releasing body fat and unwanted illness!

Chapter 1

Why Me?

During my interviewing of queasy people, somewhere in our conversation, most of them would eventually say something like: "Why me?" "Why can't I eat like so and so and never gain a pound?" That's why I decided to name this section Why Me? Indirectly, it's not your fault. As you read this masterpiece, you'll begin to see for yourself. You may also learn some things about yourself you may not have known before. All the common factors from the 200 people interviewed are 100 percent! Meaning the group of one hundred people who released weight made these changes, while the other group of one hundred people who are still queasy did not make these changes! I also noticed most of the queasy people used excuse as to why they could not make the changes instead of reasons why they should and could make the changes. One of the most profound statements I've ever heard was, "If you want things in your life to change, you have to change things in your life." How simple and brilliant is that statement! It's so simple that most of you will let it go in one ear and out the other!

Now, the "why me." Why? Because you are you. Your body responds differently than so and so's does when that person consumes the same thing you consume. For example, we've all seen a person consume a countless number of alcoholic beverages and not seem affected, while another person can consume a small amount of the same alcoholic beverage and be hammered. That should answer the question "why me." This also should explain why a certain diet program may work for one person and not another.

What am I consuming?

RIP

Marilyn Marlene Booker

I love you and I miss you more than words can say.

My sister was called home at the tender age of thirty-six. She was diagnosed with cancer. I cried and prayed more than I ever had in my life. I kept asking God, "How can this happen to my sister? Why did my parents have to lose a child? How did my sister DEVELOP cancer?" And God answered me!

A wise man investigates what a fool takes for granted!

Matthew 7:7–8 (KJ21)

Ask and it shall be given you; seek, and ye shall find; knock, and it shall be opened unto you. For everyone that asketh receiveth; and he that seeketh findeth; and him that knocketh it shall be opened.

My sister departed the universe on November 29, 2005.
Approximately one month before her passing, I was introduced to a company named Tahitian Noni. Noni is a fruit that comes from the *Morinda citrifolia* Tree and is indigenous to Southeast Asia, the Pacific, and Caribbean. Noni has a rich history dating back thousands of years. It is believed to be God's Gift. It is used as a remedy for

many ailments, including cancer. Many people call noni juice "the magic juice."

I was very intrigued by this company. It was a network marketing opportunity. So I became a business partner with the company. I paid my dues and fees and ordered two cases of the noni juice. One night, during my anxious anticipation of my shipment, I woke a little past 3:00 a.m. to my sister Marlene banging on my door and yelling my name. As I awoke, I was sweating, and I felt extremely sad. I rushed down the stairs to open the door for her. When I opened the door, no one was there. I immediately knew I was dreaming. I sat on the couch and began to weep. I wanted to call a few family members to explain what I was going through, but instantly said to myself no one would understand. So I did the only thing I thought I could do at the time to lift me up, I smoked a blunt! As I put the roach in the ashtray, I laid back on the couch and stretched out. When I put my feet up, the heel of my right foot pressed the remote control and the TV cut on. I didn't even think about cutting it off, I just closed my eyes and began to breathe deeply. All of a sudden, I hear a very passionate voice claiming natural cures for any and every disease, including cancer. Now, I dreaded those damned late-night TV infomercials. But I popped up like ready toast in a toaster. I didn't think twice about picking up the phone and ordering this book. The book was *Natural Cures "They" Don't Want You to Know About* by Kevin Trudeau, and of course, I requested the two-day shipping option. The book arrived a day before the Noni shipment. I was appalled at what I read. I highly recommend you read that book. It will blow your mind.

I decided to bring a case of noni juice to my next visit with my sister, and I was armed with an arsenal of questions for the doctors. A nurse came in to give her something. I asked what it was, and the nurse replied with an answer and the reason for the drug. I offered my two cents before she gave her the drug. At her own choice, she didn't give her the drug and instead left the room. Three doctors returned and asked my parents and I to come with them for a discussion. The first question one of the doctors asked me was if I was into health care. I replied, "What do you mean?"

Another doctor answered, "Are you a health care practitioner?"

I was offended by the questions and got angry, basically asking, "Why aren't you all trying these other methods that have been proven to work for other patients around the world?"

And their answer was basically,
"Only an approved drug can cure,
treat, and/or prevent a disease." I
was also instructed to calm down or
I would be removed from the
hospital. About a week later,
Marlene was transferred to hospice,
and you know what happens after
that.

During the preparation for the
arrangements, all I could talk about
was the information I had read in
the *Natural Cures* book and this
magic juice. Nobody understood. I
showed the book to people, but
nobody read it. I was baffled. The
day had arrived for me to take the
information for the obituary to the
family who had offered to design
and finalize it. As soon as I sat

down at the computer with her, I noticed a case of noni juice sitting on the floor. I eagerly explained I had just become a distributor with Tahitian Noni, and I mentioned the information in the *Natural Cures* book. I talked so much, and all she did was listen, nodding her head in agreement and murmuring "mm-hmm."

She never said anything except questions and comments about the obituary. As I was leaving, her dad said, "Sugarman, sit down for a minute." Before I could get comfortable on the couch, he said to me, "Sugarman, you are absolutely right about everything I just heard you say. I know because I was diagnosed with cancer a short while ago, and instead of the drugs and surgery, I began drinking noni juice, completely changed my diet, and did a few other natural treatments and remedies. Today, I am cancer free!"

I never knew that:

Virtually everything we put in our mouths and on our skin has man-made drugs and chemicals in it. The FDA has reportedly approved and allowed somewhere around 15,000 of these drugs and chemicals to be used in the food and products we buy and use daily, including tap water! The scary part is most of these drugs and chemicals don't have to be put on the labels or listed in the ingredients. A perfect example of this is cigarettes. We all know cigarettes are bad for us. But the makers of cigarettes don't have to list a single ingredient on the package! This is insane! These companies don't have to tell us they are loading us with these man-made drugs and chemicals because the FDA says it's OK. The moment I was told this, I wanted to know more.

My need to know has always been greater than my desire to be fooled. I wanted to know what these drugs and chemicals were, and the effect these drugs and chemicals have on the human body. Up to that point in my life, I'd never worried about what I was eating, drinking, or putting on my skin.

Here's a few examples
presented to me:

-Most meats come from animals
that have been genetically
modified and fed in an unnatural
way. They have also been
injected with growth hormones,
antibiotics, and other drugs.

-Most fruits and vegetables are
loaded with herbicides,
pesticides, insecticides, etc.
They are manufactured in
warehouses, not grown on
farms.

-Cosmetics and cleaning
products have deadly chemicals
listed in the ingredients.

-Some drugs and chemicals may be listed as "SPICE" or "SPICES." This was approved by the FDA.

-Tap water is loaded with drugs and chemicals including fluoride and chlorine.

-Farm-raised fish is loaded with chemicals and drugs.

-Homogenized and pasteurized products, hydrogenated oils, trans fats, margarine, and chlorinated water may be extremely harmful and may cause illnesses.

-White sugar and white flour could cause insulin secretion and have us in a diabetic state.

-Every person with a disease (cancer, diabetes, heart disease, obesity, etc.) eat fast food, restaurant food, and other processed foods.

-Toothpaste with FLUORIDE has a warning that says "If accidentally swallowed, get medical help or contact a POISON CONTROL CENTER RIGHT AWAY!"

WOW

See, it was obvious that God answered my prayers and revealed to me the CAUSE of my sister's cancer.

If a person is consuming all these man-made drugs and chemicals every day, it could increase their chances of DEVELOPING a disease or obesity.

This is about releasing weight, so let's talk about fat. You'll notice I will not make statements like "weight loss" or "losing weight" simply because when we lose something, subconsciously, we try to find it. Also, you have to stop saying and thinking about being overweight. Rather, focus your thoughts and statements on being thin. Don't say or think about eliminating food cravings, focus on having a normal appetite. Here's a few examples of some positive thoughts you can use daily:

I have the power to reclaim the body weight I had when I was so and so age.

In a short amount of time, I will look the way I looked in this picture.

I'm beginning to feel more at ease about my body weight.

I've discovered this process to be easier than anything ever before.

My physical body is coming into alignment with my dream body.

My metabolism is cooperating with me much more.

Wouldn't it be nice if the food burning characteristics of my body kicked into a higher gear and this turned into an easy and almost effortless process.

I'm feeling a greater inspiration to exercise.

I know the results won't be instant, but the right me is coming into being in its perfect time.

Always put your thoughts and

statements in the affirmative!
Focus on what you want, not
what you don't want!

The human body has three
kinds of fat.

The first is structural fat, which
surrounds the joints and organs.

The second is normal fat
reserves, which is used for fuel
when the body is insufficient.

The third is abnormal fat
reserves, also for fuel.

The first two are needed for

good health.

The third is located in the problem areas: Hips, buttocks, thighs, triceps area, ankles, stomach, neck, waist, etc. This third fat will release during pregnancy to help feed the fetus and in severe nutritional emergencies. Another way to say nutritional emergency is **starvation!**

The human body is designed with seventy-eight organs that need to function properly in order to have optimum health. Organs consist of millions of cells. Each organ has a different size, shape, and function. Certain groups of organs are essential for one function.

Some of these organs are glands.

Our bodies have two types of glands.

Exocrine glands and endocrine glands.

Exocrine glands secrete their product into duct channels that carry them either to the outside of the body or into body cavities.

Endocrine glands produce hormones that regulate metabolism, growth and development, tissue function, sexual function, fat distribution, reproduction, sleep, mood, appetite, and a few other things.

Here is a list of a few of these vitally important glands:

Endocrine:
-Hypothalamus
-Pituitary (anterior and posterior)
-Adrenal
-Thyroid
-Gonads
-Thymus
-Pancreas
-Pineal
-Prostate (male only)

Exocrine:
-Lachrymal
-Sweat
-Salivary
-Mammary (female only)
-Sebaceous
-Ceruminous

Now a list of some very important organs. These organs will be listed in order of largest to smallest:

-Skin
-Liver
-Brain
-Lungs
-Heart
-Kidneys
-Spleen
-Pancreas

Everything we put in our mouth and on our skin will determine how our organs and glands function. Our organs and glands are being overtaxed and abused. We are literally killing ourselves. Unknowingly! We are being misinformed. We are being treated like lab rats. Most of us believe we are eating healthy. Most of us trust these companies too much. Most of us believe we are healthy.

Healthy people do not have allergies, aches, and pains. Healthy people do not take drugs. A healthy person lives without illness, sickness, or disease. Healthy people do not need surgeries. Healthy people do not have skin problems. Healthy people do not feel depressed or stressed. A healthy person isn't overweight. The list goes on.

Most of us have no idea how good we can really feel. Most of us believe it's normal to get sick and/or feel discomfort. Most of us believe we have to take drugs for good health.

I believe the exact opposite to be true!

Queasy people have an anomalous hypothalamus gland! The hypothalamus gland is a very important gland. If this gland isn't operating properly, it can lead to a host of problems. This is the gland that allocates the bodies' metabolism, appetite, storing of fat, sex drive, mood, thirst, sleep, and temperature regulation. THIS GLAND MUST BE RESET AND NORMALIZED!

Here are some common problems that queasy people have, not listed in order of importance because, as mentioned, everyone is diverse.

1. The type of food they eat
2. Food cravings
3. Low metabolism
4. Intense hunger
5. Sluggish digestive system
6. A clogged liver
7. Lack of walking
8. Eating restaurant food
9. Low muscle mass
10. Eating before bed
11. Little or no breakfast
12. Lack of sweating
13. Parasites
14. Nutritional deficiencies
15. Lack of oxygen
16. Allergies
17. Heavy metal toxicity

18. Poor circulation
19. Candida yeast overgrowth
20. A clogged colon
21. Lack of enzymes
22. Hormonal imbalances
23. Underactive thyroid
24. Inept pancreas
25. Consume homogenized and pasteurized dairy
26. Affected by growth hormones in meat and dairy
27. Lack of water
28. Consume monosodium glutamate (MSG)
29. Consume artificial sweeteners
30. Consume carbonated drinks
31. Eat microwaved foods
32. Take prescription and over-the-counter drugs
33. Eat high fructose corn syrup
34. Consume fluoride
35. Their own thoughts

36. Lack of exercise

The list of problems you just read barely scratches the surface. There are other factors, and one of them could be genetics. I was told genetics play a huge role because more than likely, the child will develop many eating, thinking, and environmental habits from the people who raised him or her.

It is also believed that the list is the cause of many infirmities. All illnesses are either cultivated, incurred, or you're born with it.

Most of us are unaware of the processing techniques and all the drugs, chemicals, growth hormones, herbicides, pesticides, antibiotics, etc., that are being used in our food, cosmetics, cleaning products, and even our water supply! Our dairy and other drinks are homogenized and pasteurized!

Remember the saying:
You are what you eat

We have no idea the effect these processing techniques, drugs, and chemicals that are used are having on us. But you might have some idea now. I know you're sitting there asking why "they" are doing that to the food, other products, and water. STOP RIGHT THERE! First, ask yourself who "they" are. From now on and for the rest of your life, whenever you use that ole saying "THEY SAY," always ask yourself who are "they." Now, back to your original question. Why are "they" doing this?

Sources say the following!

-To make us fat
-To enhance taste and texture
-To preserve the food
-To increase appetite
-To give us disease
-To get us addicted

The best way for these companies to make money is to produce the product as cheaply as possible and with a long shelf life.

Another reason, and this may

upset you, is to get us fat (I used that F word because I want you to understand the significance), queasy, and addicted to the product. It's a psychological addiction! That's just a few reasons presented to me.

Read The Real Thing—The Truth & Power at The Coca Cola Company.

(This explains how cocaine was an important ingredient to get the consumers addicted!)

All the reasons have one common denominator; they increase profits!

Queasy people are great

customers for the drug and food industry.

I was told the main reason people remain sick and overweight is because they only treat their symptoms and not what's causing their symptoms.

Example:
If I stab myself with a knife, I would go to the hospital and receive "treatment" for my "symptoms." My "symptoms" would be pain and bleeding. My "treatment" would be drugs for my pain and surgery for my wound. If I continue to stab myself, I'll continue needing drugs and surgery. If I don't stop doing what's causing the problem, I'll always need

"treatment."

Now ask yourself:
What are you stabbing yourself
with?

This is kind of a straight-to-the
point book. I can give you a
bunch of stories, but screw all
that. However, there are many
references at the end of this
book. Do your own research.
After all, your health is your
responsibility. As stated, I am
not a doctor. I have no medical
training. As a researcher,
journalist, investigator, and
reporter, I'm sharing information
about possible causes of
obesity and disease. So are you
ready to start a new beginning?
Are you ready to release that

extra weight so you can become
that energetic, thin happy
person God intended you to be?
I know you are.

So let's go!

Chapter 2

30–60 Day Release

1. Do not eat any fast food or
restaurant food at all.
These restaurants produce food
in the most unnatural way. The
food is designed to taste good
but is extremely unhealthy.

2. Get fifteen colonics in 30–45

days.
There is an excellent chance
you have several pounds of
undigested fecal matter stuck in
your colon. This waste can and
will cause several problems. A
dramatic improvement could be
noticed immediately after
cleaning your colon. You must
see a licensed colon therapist.

3. Do a candida cleanse.
Candida yeast overgrowth must
be wiped out of your body.
When you wipe out candida,
you could wipe out food
cravings, allergies, hormonal
imbalances, fatigue, poor
digestion, and many other
problems.

4. Stop eating pork.

Remember you are what you eat! Dr. Jeff McCombs wrote a book called LifeForce: A Dynamic Plan for Health, Vitality, and Weight Loss. It's a must read!

5. Do a colon cleanse.
This could improve the function of all organs and glands. You could also see better looking skin, hair, and nails. You may also experience an increase in energy and metabolism.

6. Drink one-half to one gallon of water daily.
Immediately drink a large glass of water as soon as you wake up in the morning. Spring or distilled water is highly recommended. Do not drink tap

water. Tap water is loaded with chlorine, fluoride, and other contaminates. Buy filters for all faucets.

7. Walk outside one hour nonstop every day.
Only use a treadmill as a last option. Walking outside at a pace where you can maintain a conversation is extremely beneficial.

8. Use organic raw apple cider vinegar, with the mother, daily.
A tablespoon three times a day is ideal.

9. Use organic unrefined virgin coconut oil daily.
A tablespoon two times a day is ideal.

10. Take whole food
supplements.
This could help improve
nutritional deficiencies.

11. Throw your microwave
away.
Or take it to the scrap yard for a
little extra money. Research
shows that microwaved food
has an adverse effect on the
body.

12. Eat only organic food.
Ideally, you want only 100
percent organic food. The next
best is food labeled organic.
The majority of that product is
organic. The next after that is
products labeled as made with
organic ingredients. The

minority of that product is organic.

13. Absolutely no prescription or nonprescription drugs.
(Consult with your doctor.) Over-the-counter, nonprescription, and even prescription DRUGS may be your biggest problem! All are man-made!

14. Take digestive enzymes. Take with every meal. This could help dramatically improve the body's natural ability to digest food.

15. No lotions or creams on your skin.
If you can't eat it, don't put it on your skin. Most of these

products we use contain things like mineral oil, propylene glycol, sodium laurel sulfate, carbomer, phenoxyethanol, methylparaben, dimethicone, and a host of things we can't even pronounce.

16. Eat two or more organic apples every day.
Remember the saying, "An apple a day keeps the doctor away." Apples could help regulate blood sugar, reduce appetite, and help clean the liver, gallbladder, and colon.

17. Eat two or more organic grapefruits every day.
Grapefruit has enzymes that could help release fat and reduce food cravings.

18. Add coral calcium daily. Calcium supplementation could have major health benefits, including losing weight. Most people are deficient in calcium.

19. Drink one cup or more of organic green tea daily. This tea could regulate hunger, increase metabolism, and stimulate cleansing of the cells.

20. Drink one cup or more of organic yerba mate tea. This tea could increase energy, stimulate the releasing of fat cells, and reduce appetite.

21. Drink one cup or more of organic chamomile tea daily. This tea could help relax the

body completely.

22. Drink one cup or more of organic Eleotin tea daily.
This tea could extremely improve the function of the pancreas.

23. Take probiotics.
This could improve digestion, help with cleansing, and stimulate metabolism.

24. Eat a large breakfast daily.
Research shows most overweight people eat little or no breakfast. Everything you eat must be organic. Adding organic hot peppers, sauce, or salsa could have a huge benefit in helping to increase metabolism and reducing your appetite.

25. Take Acetyl L-Carnitine.
This amino acid could help turn fat into fuel and increase metabolic rate. It could also benefit muscle tissue.

26. Eat protein before you go to bed.
One hundred grams of organic beef, veal, turkey, or fish could help stimulate the mobilization of fat cells and decrease water retention, promoting the burning of fat while sleeping.

27. Eat dinner before 6:00 p.m.
Three and a half hours before you go to sleep is what's recommended.

28. Eat six times a day.

This can be done with breakfast, lunch, dinner, and snacks in between. Try not to eat anything after 7:00 p.m.

29. Use organic cinnamon as often as possible.
Organic cinnamon could help regulate blood sugar and insulin. Cinnamon could also help release fat reserves and normalize appetite.

30. Eat organic hot peppers.
Eating these peppers could help reduce appetite and increase metabolism. They could also be great at helping release fat. Anything such as hot salsas and hot sauce should be used as much as possible.

31. Eat a 100 percent organic salad with lunch and dinner. Every vegetable and ingredient should be organic. Adding 100 percent organic extra virgin olive oil and 100 percent organic raw apple cider vinegar with the mother to salads is a bonus! This could add vital enzymes and nutrients that could stimulate the release of stored fat. The important fiber that's being added could help regulate blood sugar and appetite.

32. No farm-raised fish.
All fish you eat should be wild caught. Farm-raised fish should never be consumed.

33. Do not eat nitrites.
Eating foods with nitrites can

cause weight gain, food cravings, and hormonal imbalances.

34. Do not eat trans fats.
Trans fats can also be products like margarine! Check the ingredients for hydrogenated or partially hydrogenated oils. These are also trans fats.

35. Do not eat high fructose corn syrup.
If the ingredients say maltodextrose, dextrose, sucrose, corn syrup, or high fructose corn syrup, don't eat it.

36. No monosodium glutamate (MSG).
MSG is a flavor enhancer and preservative. It is called an

excitotoxin.

37. No artificial sweeteners.
NutraSweet, Splenda,
aspartame, sucralose, or
saccharin should never be
consumed.

38. Eliminate carbonated drinks.
These drinks can block the
absorption of calcium. They can
also adversely affect the
pancreas. Diet drinks are worse
than regular drinks. If you must
have a carbonated drink, make
sure it's organic.

39. Limit ice cold drinks.
Drinking ice cold beverages can
slow metabolism and increase
hunger.

40. Use organic natural sweeteners.
Stevia is a great option. This all-natural herb could help regulate blood sugar and stimulate weight loss. Other options are organic agave nectar, raw organic honey, or raw organic sugar cane.

41. Sweat in a sauna.
Sweating in an infrared sauna for twenty minutes a day may be hard because of our busy schedules, but it's highly recommended.

42. Get more sun.
The sun is the best source of vitamin D.

43. Use krill oil.

Taking this supplement could increase circulation and oxygen in the body. It could be extremely beneficial to the liver and pancreas.

44. Get proper sleep.
10:00 p.m. to 6:00 a.m. is the ideal sleep times. Between 11:00 p.m. and 2:00 a.m., the body releases certain healing hormones. Being asleep during these hours could improve your health.

45. Take vitamin E.
The right all-natural vitamin E could improve liver and gallbladder function. It can be a powerful boost for weight loss, beautiful looking skin, and for keeping the arteries open.

46. Add fiber.
Fiber could increase digestion, relieve constipation, and help cleanse the body.

47. Jump on a mini-trampoline (rebounder) daily.
(rebounder)
Jumping on this for five to ten minutes daily could have miraculous physical and mental health benefits. You will be amazed with the results!

48. Get massages regularly.
As much as possible, get a massage. A minimum of three per week is recommended.

49. Eliminate deodorants and antiperspirants.

Aluminum zirconium tetrachlorohydrex gly, cyclopentasiloxane, and all the other poisons we can't pronounce should be avoided at all costs.

50. Buy a shower filter.
The skin in the largest organ. The chemicals in tap water are absorbed and can be extremely harmful to the body.

51. Reduce air conditioning.
People who spend more time in air conditioning could gain weight easier and faster than people who spend less time in air conditioning.

52. Reduce fluorescent lights.
Fluorescent light may cause

chemical reactions in the brain that cause fatigue and depression, leading to food cravings.

53. Use electromagnetic chaos eliminators.
Use of these items could increase energy, give better mental clarity, and create better functioning of the body.

54. Practice deep breathing multiple times daily.
Use your lungs. Inhale four seconds, exhale four seconds. This could increase oxygen in the body. Believe it or not, most of us are deficient in oxygen.

55. Do a heavy metal cleanse. This could improve circulation,

energy, and metabolism.

Doing as much as possible on this list for the 30–60 day period will be your first step in eliminating fat and harmful toxins from the body. You could also be dramatically improving the natural functions of your organs and glands. The amount of weight released depends on the individual. Most individuals release one pound per day.

Chapter 3

21–45 Day Release

This must be done under the supervision of a licensed health care practitioner!

Hundreds of thousands of people around the world used this weight loss protocol discovered by A.T.W. Simeon, MD. You absolutely must read his book Pounds and Inches: A New Approach to Obesity. This protocol requires daily injections of hCG (human chorionic gonadotropin). hCG is a natural substance that is produced in the female body during pregnancy. This substance is extracted from the urine of pregnant women. It is then purified and made into pharmaceutical grade hCG. Although hCG is a natural substance, it is classified as a drug! So it is only available with a prescription. If your doctor refuses to prescribe hCG to you, find another doctor!

The Simeon weight loss protocol requires daily injection of hCG combined with a very specific eating plan.

Because I'm not a doctor, the injections will not be printed in this book.

For informational purposes, here are the specific foods to eat.

Day 1

*Eat whatever you want as described in step 1. Eat as much organic food as you like.

*Drink one-half half to one gallon of spring or distilled water with coral calcium sachets throughout the day.

Day 2

*Repeat day 1.

Day 3–21 (up to 45)

*Drink one-half to one gallon of spring or distilled water with coral calcium sachets throughout the day.

*For breakfast only have:
black coffee, or
green tea, or
yerba mate tea, or
Wu Long tea, or
chamomile tea.

You may drink as much of the teas as you like. Never make your tea or coffee with tap water.

*For lunch and dinner only have:
100 grams of:
organic grass-fed beef or veal,
or
organic chicken breast, or
wild Chilean sea bass, or
flounder, or
sole, or
halibut.

Ideally, these meats should be grilled. Bake them if you can't grill them. Do not use oils or fats.

One large handful of one of the

following organic vegetables:
asparagus
chard
celery
beet greens
cabbage
cucumbers
red radishes
white, yellow, or red onions
fennel
tomatoes
spinach
lettuces of any kind

Vegetables can be eaten raw, steamed, grilled, or gently boiled. You can season your food with organic herbs of any kind. Organic sea salt, juice squeezed from half of an organic lemon, organic raw apple cider vinegar, or organic black pepper. Absolutely no oils, butter, or dressings.

One organic apple, organic grapefruit, or some organic strawberries can be eaten during or between meals.

Drink as much of the teas, coffee, or water as you like. Remember, never use tap water.

Never have two of the exact same meals in the same day. Lunch and dinner must be two different meals.

This step must be done a minimum of 21 days, a maximum of 45 days. The specific foods used could cause chemical reactions in the body, and combined with the hCG, activate the hypothalamus into releasing the secure abnormal fat reserves.

If hCG is completely unavailable to you, then replace step 2 with:

The Turbo Protein Diet written by Dieter Markert.
This protocol uses a product called
Almased.

For the change seekers who have made it this far, I know you're smiling from ear to ear, and experiencing some miraculous benefits. I know you may also be upset and maybe even furious about how you have been misled and treated like your life doesn't matter. But good always trumps evil!

Chapter 4

21–30 Day Release

This should be followed for 21–30 days, while doing some of the things in step 1. You can eat anything you like, with the following exceptions:

For 21–30 days

Step 1:
No sugar, honey, molasses, or sweetener of any kind.
No starch, including breads, pastas, potatoes, white rice, yams, or any wheat product,

etc.

In addition to doing the recommendations in step 1:

1. Drink one-half to one gallon of water daily, ideally with coral calcium sachets.

2. Take Three-Lac as directed.

3. Sit at a table and be relaxed when eating a meal.

4. Do not eat in front of a TV, in a car, or standing up.

5. Put smaller amounts of food on your plate.

6. Do a liver cleanse. Cleansing the liver could

dramatically improve digestion, increase metabolism, and promote permanent weight loss.

7. Do a parasite cleanse.
This should be done after doing a colon cleanse and liver cleanse. This could increase energy and promote weight regulation.

8. Wear magnetic finger rings.

9. Use a rebounder (mini-trampoline) for five to ten minutes daily.
This could allow you to stimulate and strengthen every cell in the body simultaneously.

10. Eliminate dairy products.

11. Walk for one hour nonstop every day.

12. Change your thoughts about yourself.
Research proves that we become what we think. Very few people understand what that means.

13. Don't watch the news.
Watching the news can fill your mind with negative pictures. This could create worry and stress.

14. Don't read the newspaper.
The newspaper can fill your mind with negative stories. These stories can create worry and stress.

15. Have sex more often.
This should be at the top of everyone's list! Sex could promote excellent health!

16. Don't eat anything that has one of the following on the label: low carbs
fat free
diet
sugar free
etc.

17. Do not use nonstick cookware.
Teflon nonstick cookware could be extremely harmful.

18. Exercise more often.
There are seven basic forms of exercise that you should participate in. Here they are:

A. stretching
B. resistance
C. posture
D. slow rhythmic movement
E. aerobic
F. anaerobic
G. cellular

19. Eat raw organic nuts and seeds.
Stay away from roasted and salted nuts and seeds. Try to buy them still in a shell; they retain more nutrients.

20. Get a chiropractic adjustment.
Many of us have a misaligned spine. Do this once a month.

It's recommended that you weigh yourself every morning

after emptying your bladder. If you notice more than two pounds gained during this process, stop consumption of all food and only drink water until 6:00 p.m. that day. You can also drink the recommended teas, and you may use stevia in the teas as your sweetener. At about 6:15 p.m., eat the biggest organic grass-fed steak you can. Any organic grass-fed beef will do. No salt should be added; season it with organic herbs and peppers. Eat an organic tomato or apple with it.

Weigh yourself again; if your weight is the same, repeat that process. It's highly recommended you repeat this process for two days.

You should be releasing a pound a day. That's why it's important to weigh yourself daily.

Chapter 5

A New Beginning

Eliminating toxins that have built up in our systems is vitally important.

Here is a list of some cleanses:
- A. colon cleanse
- B. liver cleanse
- C. gallbladder cleanse
- D. lung cleanse
- E. fat tissue cleanse
- F. lymphatic system cleanse
- G. heavy metal cleanse

H. parasite cleanse
I. candida cleanse
J. full body cleanse

Doing these cleanses could have a dramatic benefit for multiple conditions, including releasing extra weight. Studies show these cleanse can improve the function of the human body better than any man-made drug. In most cases, after doing the cleanses, you could eliminate every single illness! The reason your doctor hasn't told you about these cleanses could be because he or she needs you as a customer for the rest of your life. A healthy person doesn't need doctors! By the way, the cleanses are not drugs!!

Research shows weight gain, in most cases, may not be caused by calories, fat, complex or simple carbohydrates, high glycemic rated foods, or sodium. Obesity and weight gain could be caused by NONPRESCRIPTION AND PRESCRIPTION DRUGS, MAN-MADE INGREDIENTS, DRUGS, AND CHEMICALS IN COSMETICS, WATER, AND FOOD. ALSO THE FOOD PROCESSING TECHNIQUES EMPLOYED IN THE GROWING, PRODUCING, AND MANUFACTURING OF FOOD!

EAT 100 percent ORGANIC FOOD!

If it's not 100 percent organic, make sure it's ORGANIC!

Use organic cosmetic and cleaning products!

Here's the Holy Health Tabulations:

See various natural health care practitioners and/or providers on a regular basis.

Read all the books, watch all the documentaries, call the phone numbers, and go to the websites recommended.

Don't eat any fast food or restaurant food. Absolutely none.

Stop taking nonprescription and prescription drugs.
(Consult with your doctor before doing this.)

Buy a juice machine and make your own juice.

Check your body's pH.

Get natural sunlight on a regular basis.

Do all the cleanses listed.

Only eat organic fruits and vegetables.

Avoid Propylene sulfate.

Don't drink tap water.

Do alphabiotics.

Buy a shower filter and filters for every faucet.

Take coral calcium.

Wear magnetic toe and finger rings.

Do energetic rebalancing.

Eat one organic apple every day.

Use a rebounder daily.

Take whole food supplements daily.

Only eat organic meat and poultry.

Sleep on a magnetic mattress pad.

Limit bottled and canned juice.

Get colonics as needed.

Walk outside more often.

Avoid sodium laurel sulfate.

See an herbalist.

See a chiropractor.

Don't consume MSG.

Don't consume aspartame.

Don't consume high fructose corn syrup.

Do chi kung.

See a homeopathic practitioner.

Use foot orthotics.

Eat snacks.

Reduce TV time.

Avoid diethanolamine (DEA).

Don't watch the news.

Don't read the newspaper.

Plant a garden.

Cook on a regular basis.

Don't use an alarm clock.

Use aromatherapy.

Commit countless acts of kindness.

Make your own wine and beer.

Don't use corn oil.

Eliminate or reduce air conditioning.

Eliminate air fresheners.

Use full spectrum lights.

Sleep eight hours.

Do tai chi.

Drink the magic juices.
Noni, Zija, pomegranate,
mangosteen, MonaVie, goji,
aloe vera, acai berry,
FrequenSea.

Get a pet.

Eat organic dark chocolate.

Get an inversion table.

Get out of debt.

Get a range motion machine.

Get rolfing.

*Use the Callahan techniques
on a regular basis.*

Listen to good music.

Put living plants in your home.

Laugh often.

Lift weights.

Be thankful.

Don't drive and use a cell phone at the same time.

Be lighthearted.

Get massages regularly.

Get and give hugs daily.

Stretch the tendons and muscles in your body daily.

Stop smoking.

Find your purpose in life.

Drink eight full glasses of water daily.

Drive less.

Do not eat food bars.

Take omega-3 supplements.

Use organic sea salt.

Do a seven- to thirty-day fast.

Smile all day.

Do dianetics/scientology.

Fast on occasion.

Don't eat after 7:00 p.m.

Avoid swimming pools, steam rooms, and hot tubs.

Don't eat white processed sugar.

Give yourself a dry-brush massage often.

Don't eat white processed flour.

Avoid anything that has low carbs, fat free, sugar free, healthy, light, and all natural on the label if it's not organic.

Stop eating pork.

Stop eating farm-raised fish.

Stop eating shellfish.

Only eat wild caught fish.

Get an air purifier.

Don't eat or drink pasteurized and homogenized dairy products.

Don't eat hydrogenated or partially hydrogenated oils (trans fats).

Speak positive words and statements.

Don't eat food that comes in a box, can, or package.

*Don't use sun block or
sunscreen.*

Get an oxygen water cooler.

Listen to destressing CDs.

*Don't consume any artificial
sweeteners.*

Sweat on a regular basis.

*Neutralize electromagnetic
chaos.*

*Get treated by a bio energetic
synchronization technique
practitioner.*

*Eat organic raw seeds and nuts
for snacks.*

Practice deep breathing every day.

Don't use skin products you can't eat.

Exercise on a regular basis.

Use a gentle wind project instrument.

Don't use deodorants or antiperspirants with aluminum.

Stop using florescent lights.

Rest from Friday sundown to Saturday sundown.

*Don't take vitamin

supplements.*

Go to sleep at 10:00 p.m. and wake up at 6:00 a.m.

Wear white often.

Take a short break in the afternoon.

Write goals down on white paper with blue ink.

Use organic apple cider vinegar with the mother daily.

Use organic unrefined virgin coconut oil daily.

Avoid brand name products.

*Use toothpaste without

fluoride.*

Only use organic cleaning products.

Buy a vacuum cleaner with a HEPA filter.

Use liquid colloidal minerals daily.

Avoid psychiatrists and psychologists.

Address nutritional deficiencies.

This is your new life. This is the way God intended us to be. God did not create us to be slaves to these companies. God did not intend for us to be full of drugs and chemicals. If our bodies are going to be filled with things God didn't create, it should be by our choice, not the corporations that are selling us food, cosmetics, and other products. I remember "people" used to be called "humanity," "individuals," "public at large," or "citizens." Now I hear these corporations, and even our government, refer to us as "CONSUMERS." Fast-food executives refer to customers who eat fast food once a week as "HEAVY USERS."

Educate yourself! Know what's going on and what's being done to you and, more importantly, our children. Don't leave it up to doctors, priests, hospitals, schools, or anyone else. It's your life.

TAKE COMPLETE CONTROL!

Chapter 6

You Must Read Labels and Ingredients

There are many toxic drugs and chemicals in the majority of the food we eat in restaurants and buy from the supermarket. The food supply is very different than it was some years ago. The food nowadays is being produced the cheapest way possible. The man-made drugs and chemicals being added and the processing techniques destroy the living beneficial enzymes in the food, wiping out much of its nutritional value.

Avoid all restaurants! Avoid all supermarkets! Shop at health food stores, farmers' markets, and whole food stores! Avoid brand name products and/or publicly traded food companies! Read the label first, then the ingredients! Here's a quick review of some of the things you should avoid:

-Saccharin
-Palm oil
-Dextrose
-Mineral oil
-Sucrose
-Soy protein isolate
-Monosodium glutamate (MSG)

-Aspartame
-Propylene glycol
-High fructose corn syrup
-Hydrogenated or partially hydrogenated oil of any kind (trans fats)
-Natural and/or artificial flavors
-Artificial colors
-Enriched bleached flour of any kind
-Sucralose—Splenda
-Sodium laureth sulfate
-Anything you can't pronounce
-Spices
-Low carbs
-Fat free
-Diet
-Sugar free

Go to your kitchen and cosmetics cabinet now and start reading the labels and ingredients of all the products you have.

Here are a few comparisons for you:
(Food manufactures may change labels and ingredients)

1. Pancake Syrup

Aunt Jemima Syrup
Ingredients:
-corn syrup
-high fructose corn syrup
-water
-cellulose gum
-caramel color
-salt
-sodium benzoate
-sorbic acid
-artificial flavors
-natural flavors
-sodium hexametaphosphate

Organic Maple Syrup
Ingredients:
-100 percent raw unprocessed,
unfiltered maple syrup

2. Potato Chips

Dan Dee Bar-B-Q
Ingredients:
-potatoes
-vegetable oil
(one or more of the following:
canola, corn, cottonseed,
safflower, soybean, sunflower)
-salt
-fructose
-sugar
-onion, garlic, tomato powders
-paprika
-torula yeast

- -spices
- -monosodium glutamate (MSG)
- -natural flavors
- -citric acid
- -spice extractives including paprika
- -caramel color

Organic Bar-B-Q Potato Chips
Ingredients:
- -organic potatoes
- -organic expeller pressed sunflower seed, safflower, and/ or canola oil
- -sea salt
- -organic cane sugar
- -organic tomato powder
- -organic onion powder
- -organic garlic powder
- -natural mesquite smoke flavor
- -organic black pepper
- -citric acid
- -organic red pepper

-extractives of paprika

3. Mayonnaise

Miracle Whip
Ingredients:
-water
-soybean oil
-modified food starch
-high fructose corn syrup

-sugar

-salt
-contains less than 2 percent of
egg yolks
-cellulose gel
-mustard flour
-artificial color
-potassium sorbate

-xanthan gum
-cellulose gum
-spice
-paprika
-sucralose and acesulfame
potassium as sweeteners
-natural flavor
-dried garlic

Organic Mayonnaise
Ingredients:
-expeller pressed soybean oil
-organic whole eggs
-water
-organic egg yolk
-organic honey
-organic white vinegar
-sea salt
-organic dry mustard
-organic lemon juice
concentrate

4. Ketchup

Heinz Ketchup
Ingredients:
-tomato concentrate

-distilled vinegar
-high fructose corn syrup
-corn syrup
-salt
-spice
-onion powder
-natural flavors

Organic Ketchup
Ingredients:
-organic tomato paste
-organic distilled white vinegar
-water
-organic cane sugar

-organic sea salt
-organic onion
-organic allspice
-organic clove

You don't have to be super smart to know the healthier options. I can do hundreds of comparisons like this. You absolutely must read the labels and ingredients. When you begin to shop wisely, you'll be buying food that:

-will not make you fat
-will not make you addicted to the product
-tastes better
-have a lot FEWER toxins
-have much more nutrition
-make you feel better
-will not give you bloating,

headaches, gas, constipation, etc.
-will not make you hungrier

If you want to be thin, if you want to be healthy, you must increase the amount of 100 percent organic food you consume. If it's not 100 percent organic, make sure it's organic!

Understand that just because it's in a health food store doesn't mean it's healthy. That's why it's vitally important to read labels and ingredients.

Chapter 7

Culmination

The information you've just read came from thousands of experts from around the world. There will be many proponents and also many opponents. A number of you will continue to be in denial, and those are the ones who will remain fat and sick. The non-believers will continue to have uncontrollable urges to eat when not hungry, intense food cravings, and compulsive overeating habits. The skeptics will remain programmed by the hypnotic suggestive advertisements and subliminal messages designed by the food manufacturers and restaurants.

In today's world, it's virtually impossible to eat nothing but

100 percent organic food. But you can dramatically decrease the amount of unhealthy, non-organic, toxic food you consume. You can reduce the amount of unknown man-made drugs and chemicals being added to our food, water, and products simply by buying organic and drinking filtered, spring, and distilled water. Some of you non-believers might be thinking, "I boil my tap water," but all that does is kill bacteria. The fluoride, chlorine, and other unknown chemicals are still there! Buy water filters for your home. Most of you doubters will continue to take your pain relievers, cough suppressants, allergy meds, sleep aids, cold and flu meds, etc. Go right ahead; it's your own body and

health. Nobody other than you is responsible for your well-being. But if you end up with a condition and have to be rushed to the ER, don't be surprised when the doctors and nurses tell you they don't know the cause of your problems and say, "We hope this treatment works for you."

Most of you will be like those who continue to smoke cigarettes, saying, "We all have to die from something." Go ahead. It's your life. If you choose to continue to eat farm-raised fish, fast food, restaurant food, and other processed genetically modified food that's frozen, in a can, box, or package, it's your own free will. Think about this, though—you

can't catch obesity, cancer,
diabetes, high blood pressure,
heart attacks, constipation, acid
reflux, headaches, fibromyalgia,
back pain, arthritis, impotence,
low sex drive, diarrhea,
psoriasis, seizures, hair loss,
halitosis, gout, indigestion,
gastritis, migraines, gallstones,
acne, allergies, Alzheimer's,
anxiety disorder,
atherosclerosis, attention deficit
disorder (ADD/ADHD), benign
prostatic hypertrophy (BPH),
cystitis, boils, cataracts,
parasitic infection, cellulite,
chronic fatigue syndrome (CFS),
cirrhosis of the liver, congestive
heart failure, Crohn's disease,
dandruff, mastitis, depression,
eczema, osteoarthritis (OS),
emphysema, endometriosis,
fibrocystic breast, uterine

fibroids (uterine myomas), gastritis, glaucoma, hemorrhoids, Hodgkin's disease, hyperthyroidism, yeast infection, vitiligo, stress, varicose veins, restless legs syndrome, premenstrual syndrome (PMS), peptic ulcer, vaginosis, stroke, Parkinson's disease, lymphedema, lupus, kidney stones, hemochromatosis, irritable bowel syndrome, insomnia, infertility, hypothyroidism, etc. These conditions are DEVELOPED! And one of the roads that will lead you to DEVELOPMENT of a disease is through repetition of consuming something your body can't handle.

I don't believe God created our

bodies to consume countless amounts of man-made drugs and chemicals. Every time I read my Bible, I can't find a single drug or chemical. Only plants, herbs, oils, wine, and water. I've never read about doctors in the Bible. Only physicians. And my translation of "physician" is "healer." Even my Lord and Savior Jesus refused a pain relieving drink while dying on the cross. The choice is yours. Only you can decide what to put in your body. Only you can decide what to put on your skin. Some of you are thinking everyone is not meant to be skinny. Maybe that's true, but I believe no one is meant to be sick and overweight. I also believe the only reason a human is sick and overweight is by breaking the Laws of God. We must obey the Commandments. Not just the Ten Commandments, but also the Laws in the books of Exodus and Deuteronomy.

Exodus 15:26 (KJ21)
"If thou wilt diligently hearken to the voice of the Lord thy God, and wilt do that which is right in His sight, and wilt give ear to His commandments and keep all His statutes, I will put none of these diseases upon thee which I have brought upon the Egyptians; for I am the Lord that healeth thee."

Here are some additional scriptures, some of my personal

favorites, for you to research
yourself:

James 5:14–15
Matthew 6:22
Mark 11:24–25
Jeremiah 46:11
Luke 10:34
Ezekiel 47:12
Proverbs 17:22
Genesis 1:11–12
1 Timothy 5:23
Jeremiah 8:22
Matthew 21:21–22
Revelation 22:1–2
Mark 5:25–29
Genesis 1:29–30
Psalms 103:3
Romans 12:2
Exodus 23:25–26
Deuteronomy 7:15

Jeremiah 30:13

That's just a few. There are many more biblical references that can be pointed out about healing power without drugs and surgery. There were about thirty-one individual healings performed by Jesus without drugs and surgery. I've always wondered to myself how us Christians can be so sick and overweight. How can someone who claims to love Jesus be sick or overweight? And the only answer I can come up with is disobedience of the Laws.

My need to know has always been greater than my desire to be fooled!

Chapter 8

Recommended Reading

Reading books should be done on a daily basis. After high school, most of us never want to see another textbook again. If you change the way you feel about reading and read the following books listed, you could change and experience some magical benefits!

The Holy Bible

The Game of Life and How to Play It
Florence Scovel Shinn

All the Plants of the Bible
Winifred Walker

The Great American Detox Diet:
Feel Better, Look Better, and
Lose Weight by Cleaning Up
Your Diet
Alex Jamieson

Prescription for Herbal Healing:
An Easy-to-Use A-Z Reference
to Hundreds of Common
Disorders and Their Herbal
Remedies
Phyllis A. Balch CNC

Overdose: The Case Against
the Drug Companies
Jay S. Cohen, MD

Fat Land: How Americans

Became the Fattest People in the World
Greg Critser

In Tune with the Infinite
Ralph Waldo Trine

Ask and It Is Given: Learning to Manifest Your Desires
Esther and Jerry Hicks

Pounds & Inches: The Original HCG Diet Protocol
Dr. A.T.W. Simeons

Food Fight: The Inside Story of the Food Industry, America's Obesity Crisis & What We Can Do About It
Kelly D. Brownell, PhD and Katherine Battle Horgen, PhD

Mindset: The New Psychology of Success – How We Can Learn to Fulfill Our Potential
Carol S. Dweck, PhD

Sweet Deception: Why Splenda, NutraSweet, and the FDA May Be Hazardous to Your Health
Dr. Joseph Mercola and Dr. Kendra Degen Pearsall

Don't Eat This Book: Fast Food and the Supersizing of America
Morgan Spurlock

Aspartame (NutraSweet): Is It Safe?
H.J. Roberts, MD

The Hundred-Year Lie: How to Protect Yourself from the Chemicals That Are Destroying

Your Health
Randall Fitzgerald

The Disease Conspiracy: The FDA Suppression of Cures
Robert R. Barefoot

Excitotoxins: The Taste that Kills
Russell L. Blaylock, MD

The Fast Food Craze: Wreaking Havoc on Our Bodies and Our Animals
Tina Volpe

Selling Sickness: How the World's Biggest Pharmaceutical Companies Are Turning Us All Into Patients
Ray Moynihan and Alan Cassels

The End of Food: How the Food

Industry is Destroying Our Food Supply—And What We Can Do About It
Thomas F. Pawlick

No More Bull!: The Mad Cowboy Targets America's Worst Enemy: Our Diet
Howard F. Lyman with Glen Merzer & Joanna Samorow-Merzer

Trans Fats: The Hidden Killer In Our Food
Judith Shaw, MA

Hard to Swallow: The Truth about Food Additives
Doris Sarjeant and Karen Evans

Genetically Engineered Food: Changing the Nature of Nature

Martin Teitel, PhD and Kimberly A. Wilson

Our Toxic World: A Wake Up Call
Doris J. Rapp, MD

Slaughterhouse: The Shocking Story of Greed, Neglect, and Inhumane Treatment Inside the US Meat Industry
Gail A. Eisnitz

Restaurant CONFIDENTIAL: The Shocking Truth about What You're Really Eating When You're Eating Out
Michael F. Jacobson, PhD and Jayne G. Hurley, RD

Killing Cancer
Jason Winters

*New Choices in Natural Healing:
Over 1,800 of the Best Self-Help
Remedies from the World of
Alternative Medicine*
Doug Dollemore

*Rats in The Grain: The Dirty
Tricks and Trials of Archer
Daniels Midland, the
Supermarket to the World*
James B. Lieber

*Women's Intuition: Unlocking
the Wisdom of the Body*
Paula M. Reeves, PhD

Think and Grow Rich
Napoleon Hill

*The Crazy Makers: How the
Food Industry is Destroying Our*

Brains and Harming Our Children
Carol Simontacchi

The Magic of Thinking Big
David J. Schwartz, PhD

Chew On This: Everything You Don't Want to Know About Fast Food
Eric Schlosser & Charles Wilson

How to Stop Worrying and Start Living: Time-Tested Methods for Conquering Worry
Dale Carnegie

Successful Aging
John Wallis Rowe, MD and Robert Louis Kahn

Poisoned Chickens Poisoned

Eggs: An Inside Look at the Modern Poultry Industry
Karen Davis, PhD

Clear Body Clear Mind: The Effective Purification Program
L. Ron Hubbard

As a Man Thinketh
James Allen

Internal Cleansing: Rid Your Body of Toxins to Naturally and Effectively Fight Heart Disease, Chronic Pain, Fatigue, PMS, and Menopause Symptoms
Linda Berry, DC, CCN

How to Cleanse and Detoxify Your Body Today
Elson M. Haas, MD

See You at The Top
Zig Ziglar

The Amazing Liver Cleanse: A Powerful Approach to Improve Your Health and Vitality
Andreas Moritz

Don't Drink Your Milk: New Frightening Medical Facts About the World's Most Overrated Nutrient
Frank A. Oski, MD

Stopping The Clock: Why Many of Us Will Live Past 100 and Enjoy Every Minute!
Dr. Ronald Klatz and Dr. Robert Goldman

1001 All-Natural Secrets to a Pest-Free Property

Dr. Myles H. Bader

LifeForce: A Dynamic Plan for Health, Vitality, and Weight Loss
Jeffrey S. McCombs, DC

Milk: The Deadly Poison
Robert Cohen

Bitter Pills: Inside the Hazardous World of Legal Drugs
Stephen Fried

The XO Factor: Homogenized Milk May Cause Your Heart Attack
Kurt A. Oster, MD and Donald J. Ross, PhD

The Fluoride Deception
Christopher Bryson

Food Politics: How the Food Industry Influences Nutrition and Health
Marion Nestle

The Cancer Conspiracy: Betrayal, Collusion and the Suppression of Alternative Cancer Treatments
Barry Lynes

Fast Food Nation: The Dark Side of the All-American Meal
Eric Schlosser

The Drinking Water Book: How to Eliminate Harmful Toxins from Your Water
Colin Ingram

The Cancer Industry

Ralph W. Moss, PhD

Water Wasteland: Ralph Nader's Study Group Report on Water Pollution
David Zwick and Marcy Benstock

Flood Your Body with Oxygen: Therapy for Our Polluted World
Ed McCabe

Your Body's Many Cries for Water
F. Batmanghelidj, MD

How to Fight Cancer & Win
William L. Fischer

Alkalize or Die: Superior Health Through Proper Alkaline-Acid Balance

Dr. Theodore A. Baroody

Natural Cures "They" Don't Want You to Know About
Kevin Trudeau

Sowing The Wind: A Report from Ralph Nader's Center for Study of Responsive Law on Food Safety and the Chemical Harvest
Harrison Wellford

The Chemical Feast: Ralph Nader's Study Group Report on the Food and Drug Administration
James S. Turner

Healing with Magnets
Gary Null, PhD

AIDS: What the Government Isn't Telling You
Lorraine Day, MD

Dianetics: The Modern Science of Mental Health
L. Ron Hubbard

Fluoride, The Aging Factor: How to Recognize and Avoid the Devastating Effects of Flouride
Dr. John Yiamouyannis

In Bad Taste: The MSG Symptom Complex
George R. Schwartz, MD

Tapping The Healer Within: Using Thought Field Therapy to Instantly Conquer Your Fears, Anxieties, and Emotional Distress

Roger J. Callahan, PhD with Richard Trubo

Dynamic Health: Using Your Own Beliefs, Thoughts, and Memory to Create a Healthy Body
M.T. Morter

The Liver Cleansing Diet
Dr. Sandra Cabot

Rebounding to Better Health
Linda Brooks

The Miracle of Fasting: Proven Throughout History for Physical, Mental & Spiritual Rejuvenation
Paul Chappuis Bragg and Patricia Bragg

Bottom Line's Power Aging: The

Revolutionary Program to Control the Symptoms of Aging Naturally
Gary Null, PhD

Never an Outbreak: The New Breakthrough Method that Stops the Herpes Virus and Eliminates All Outbreaks
William Fharel

The Safe Shopper's Bible: A Consumer's Guide to Nontoxic Household Products, Cosmetics, and Food
David Steinman & Samuel S. Epstein, MD

Ephedra Fact & Fiction: How Politics, the Press, and Special Interests are Targeting Your Rights to Vitamins, Minerals,

and Herbs
Mike Fillon

A Shot in The Dark: Why the P in the DPT Vaccine May Be Hazardous to Your Child's Health
Harris Livermore Coulter and Barbara Loe Fisher

The Cancer Cure That Worked: Fifty Years of Suppression
Barry Lynes

Inventing The AIDS Virus
Peter H. Duesberg

The Book of Magnet Healing: A Holistic Approach to Pain Relief
Roger Coghill

Restoring Your Digestive

Health: How the Guts and Glory Program Can Transform Your Life
Jordan S. Rubin, NMD and Joseph Brasco, MD

The Big Fix: How the Pharmaceutical Industry Rips Off American Consumers
Katherine Greider

Anatomy of an Illness: As Perceived by the Patient
Norman Cousins

7 Steps to Overcoming Depression and Anxiety: A Practical Guide to Mental, Physical, and Spiritual Wellness
Gary Null

The Politics of Stupid: The Cure

for Obesity
Susan Powter

The Longevity Strategy: How to Live to 100 Using the Brain-Body Connection
David Mahoney and Richard Restak, MD

The Devil's Poison: How Flouride Is Killing You
Dean Murphy, DDS

Alternative Medicine Guide to Women's Health: Clinically Proven Alternative Therapies
Burton Goldberg

The Encyclopedia of Natural

Medicine
Michael T. Murray, ND and
Joseph Pizzorno, ND

*You Can Be…Well at Any Age:
Your Definitive Guide To Vibrant
Health & Longevity*
K. Steven Whiting, PhD

*Juice Fasting And
Detoxification: Use the Healing
Power of Fresh Juice to Feel
Young and Look Great*
Steve Meyerowitz

*The 100 Simple Secrets of
Healthy People: What Scientists
Have Learned and How You
Can Use It*
David Niven, PhD

Kidnapped: How Irresponsible

*Marketers Are Stealing the
Minds of Your Children*
Daniel S. Acuff, PhD and Robert
H. Reiher, PhD

Holocaust American Style
James R. Walker

*Politics in Healing: The
Suppression and Manipulation
of American Medicine*
Daniel Haley

*Stop The FDA: Save Your
Health Freedom*
John Morgenthaler and Steven
W. Fowkes, Editors

The Great Betrayal: Fraud in Science
Horace Freeland Judson

Leaders Are Readers!

Chapter 9

References

HAVE SOME FUN SURFING
THE NET ☺

OR
CALL TO TALK TO SOMEONE
☺

WWW.

ewater.com
800-964-4303

therawfoodworld.com
866-729-3438

nutribullet.com
800-898-8538

truealoe.com
888-440-2563

magneticosleep.com
800-265-1119

oxygenamerica.com

305-933-4219

qualityhealth.com
800-826-4148

nutiva.com
800-993-4367

citizens.org
888-774-2255

cooking.com
800-663-8810

sunorganic.com
888-269-9888

therasauna.com
888-729-7727

iahe.com
800-311-9204

acam.org
800-532-3688

ahha.org
714-779-6152

morter.com
800-874-1478

herbs.org
303-449-2265

homeopathic.com
800-359-9051

ahpa.org
301-588-1171

toolsforwellness.com
800-456-9887

reiki.com
800-332-8112

distancehealing.net
866-784-7111

frequencyrising.com
951-303-3471

i-act.org
210-366-2888

drnatura.com
800-877-0414

ejuva.com
866-463-5882

garynull.com
877-627-5065

organicconsumer.org

218-266-4164

renewlife.com
800-830-1800

abcmt.org
419-358-0273

zhenas.com
800-448-0803

naturallyfiltered.com
800-428-9419

watercuresanything.com
845-754-7866

africanredtea.com
323-658-7832

healthforce.com
800-357-2717

teaforhealth.com
855-711-1604

xango.com
877-469-2646

4spectrum.us
800-581-8906

nanocal.com
323-205-8694

qnlabs.com
800-370-3447

vites.com
888-324-9904

ota.com
802-275-3800

megafood.com
800-848-2542

drdavidwilliams.com
888-349-0483

wildernessfamilynaturals.com
800-945-3801

organic-wine.com
805-640-1255

drinklifein.com
801-494-2300

freelife.com
877-954-6244

blessedherbs.com
800-489-4372

clearbodyclearmind.com
800-722-1733

lundberg.com
530-538-3500

seaveg.com
207-412-0094

slowfoodusa.org
718-260-8000

earthsbounty.com
800-736-5609

forevergreen.org
801-655-5500

newchapter.com
800-543-7279

rockyfork.net
800-630-4534

eatwellguide.org
212-991-1930

thebrewhut.com
303-680-8898

canningpantry.com
888-858-1602

rawguru.com
800-518-0727

thewolfeclinic.com
877-359-6950

brazillivecoral.com
800-852-4064

myseaaloe.com
800-732-1150

sunrider.com
310-781-8096

4yourtype.com
877-226-8973

honeygardens.com
800-416-2083

jarrow.com
310-204-6936

melaleuca.com
800-522-3172

grassfedbeef.com
888-586-2209

oreck.com
800-219-2044

vitalchoice.com
866-482-5887

allergybegone.com
866-234-6630

ultimatelife.com
805-962-2221

sunfood.com
888-729-3663

texasgrassfedbeef.com
903-732-4653

seventhgeneration.com
800-211-4279

realgoods.com
800-919-2400

hain-celestial.com
800-434-4246

allergybuyersclub.com
888-236-7231

mdheal.org

212-989-6733

rfsafe.com
844-473-7233

burtsbees.com
800-849-7112

realmilk.com
202-363-4394

lehmans.com
800-438-5346

vitacost.com
800-381-0759

fitnessgear101.com
866-669-9320

naha.org
919-894-0298

breathdance.org
828-450-5999

theorganicpharmacy.com
310-272-7275

amoils.com
866-445-5433

feeltheqi.com
800-431-1579

promagnet.com
877-858-9082

anti-smoking.org
310-577-9828

bleedinggums.com
888-317-4402

spiritualcinemacircle.com
800-280-8290

steviasmart.com
800-577-8409

florahealth.com
800-498-3610

authenticcmo.com
800-224-8912

sldproducts.com
800-330-2563

trivita.com
800-991-7116

herbal-powers.com
877-903-9657

extendedhealth.com

800-300-6712

familyhealthnews.com
800-284-6263

aletastjames.com
212-246-2420

evolutionhealth.com
888-896-7790

hempest.com
617-412-9944

dmso.com
800-331-2638

iherb.com
951-616-3602

mysupplementstore.com
877-505-1777

alphaflex.com
775-352-2099

healthyhabits.com
800-604-6766

drwhitaker.com
888-349-0484

forcesofnaturemedicine.com
877-975-3797

healthydirections.com
888-349-0397

sambazon.com
877-726-2296

cellercise.com
866-242-2515

1healthyworld.com
315-792-1021

futurewatertoday.com
800-827-0762

gordonresearch.com
928-472-4263

www.staressence.com
888-277-4955

sunchlorellausa.com
800-829-2828

gemisphere.com
800-727-8877

patagonia.com
800-638-6464

sjaaks.com

707-775-2434

nordicnaturals.com
800-662-2544

tftrx.com
434-361-0000

rejuvenative.com
800-805-7957

barleans.com
800-445-3529

guayaki.com
888-482-9254

manukahoneyusa.com
800-395-2196

t-boost.com
866-482-6678

sourcenaturals.com
800-815-2333

pureplanet.com
800-695-2017

lef.org
800-678-8989

naet.com
714-523-8900

carlsonlabs.com
888-234-5656

twinlab.com
800-645-5626

ihealthtree.com
888-225-7778

peacefulmountain.com

888-303-3388

peelu.com
800-457-3358

natren.com
866-462-8736

naturessecret.com
800-297-3273

thecrystal.com
800-829-7625

gaiaherbs.com
888-917-8269

msm-msm.com
800-453-7516

drrons.com
877-472-8701

ysorganic.com
800-654-4593

enzymedica.com
888-918-1118

longevinex.com
866-405-4000

beealive.com
800-543-2337

thevacuumcenter.com
877-224-9998

goldminenaturalfood.com
800-475-3663

beer-wine.com
800-523-5423

eccobella.com
877-696-2220

verilux.net
800-786-6850

homebrewheaven.com
800-580-2739

heartlandmill.com
800-232-8533

1wildplanet.com
800-998-9946

eminenceorganics.com
888-747-6342

auntpattys.com
800-456-7923

petalumapoultry.com

800-556-6789

atlantafixture.com
800-282-1977

blackwing.com
800-326-7874

usa.weleda.com
800-241-1030

beyondpesticides.org
202-543-5450

lobels.com
877-783-4512

celticseasalt.com
800-867-7258

applegatefarms.com
866-587-5858

pilates.com
800-745-2837

yogafinder.com
858-213-7924

Chapter 10

Don't Believe Me, Just Watch!

For most people, listening is the easiest method of learning.

Most of the recommended readings can also be found as an audio book.

But research shows that

information obtained from reading can be much more effective.
That's why reading books is said to be magical.

Also, here are a few DVD/ Documentaries you may want to check out:

Food, Inc.

Farmageddon

The Smartest Guy in The Room

Forks Over Knives

Dallas Buyers Club

Simply Raw: Reversing Diabetes in 30 Days

Vegucated

Super Size Me

The Corporation

Food Matters

Tucker

Ingredients

Who Killed the Electric Car?

King Corn

Meet Your Meat

Prescription for Disease

The Secret

A Matter of Taste

Fat, Sick & Nearly Dead

Sister Kenny

The Constant Gardener

Iraq for Sale: The War Profiteers

Hungry for Change

Erin Brockovich

The Aviator

Chapter 11

Famous Quotes

"The greatest tragedies in the

world and personal events stem from misunderstandings." – Harvey MacKay

"Before God, we are all equally wise—and equally foolish." – Albert Einstein

"My definition of a free society is where it is safe to be unpopular." – Adlai Stevenson

"The tragedy of life is not death but what we let die inside of us while we live." – Norman Cousins

"Problems cannot be solved at the same level of awareness that created them." – Albert Einstein

"Any intelligent fool can make things bigger, more complex, and more violent. It takes a touch of genius—and a lot of courage to move in the opposite direction." – E.F. Schumacher

"You create your own universe as you go along." – Winston Churchill

"Patterning your life around others' opinions is nothing more than slavery." – Joseph Campbell

"First they ignore you, then they laugh at you, then they fight you, then you win." – An amalgamation of a speech by union leader Nicholas Klein and Mahatma Gandhi's philosophy.

"Take the first step in faith. You don't have to see the entire staircase, just take the first step." – Dr. Martin Luther King Jr.

"Orthodox medicine has not found a cure for your condition. Luckily for you I happen to be a quack."

"Whatever we think about and thank about we bring about." – John Demartini

"When you visualize, you materialize." – Dr. Denis Waitley

"[Conventional medicine is] a collection of uncertain prescriptions the results of which, taken collectively, are more fatal than useful to mankind." – Napoleon Bonaparte

"If people let the government decide what foods they eat and what medicines they take, their bodies will soon be in a sorry state as are the souls who live under tyranny." – Thomas Jefferson

"All we are is the result of our own thoughts." – attributed to Buddha

"Half of the modern drugs should be thrown out the window, except that the birds might eat them." – Dr. Martin Henry Fisher

"You don't know what you don't know."

"All truth passes through three stages. First it is ridiculed. Second it is violently opposed. Third it is accepted as self-evident." – Arthur Schopenhauer

"Whatever the mind can conceive and believe it can achieve." – Napoleon Hill

"If you think you can, or you think you can't, either way you are right." – Henry Ford

"Nearly all men can stand adversity. If you want to test a man's character give him power." – Abraham Lincoln

"Shut the iron doors on the past and the future. Live in day-tight compartments." – Dale Carnegie

"Great spirits have always encountered violent opposition from mediocre minds." – Albert Einstein

"Power tends to corrupt and absolute power corrupt absolutely." – Lord Acton

"Count your blessing not your troubles." – William Penn

"If I had my life to live over, I'd dare to make more mistakes next time." – Nadine Stair

"Prayer is the most powerful form of energy one can generate." – Alexis Carrel

"Ask for unbiased, helpful, constructive criticism." – Dale Carnegie

"Once the media touches a story the facts are lost forever." – Norman Mailer

"Who is rich? He who is content. Who is that? Nobody." – Benjamin Franklin

"Health is a state of complete physical, mental, and social well-being and not merely the absence of disease and infirmity." – The World Health Organization

"Unjust criticism is often a disguised compliment." – Dale

Carnegie

"Worry is the misuse of imagination." – Unknown

"The thing that bugs me is that people think the FDA is protecting them. It isn't. The FDA is protecting the profits of the corporations that pay us and the politicians." – Herbert Ley, MD

"To know and not to do is not to know." – Unknown

"A hospital is no place to be sick." – Samuel Goldwyn

"Happiness is not a state to arrive at, but rather a manner of traveling." – Margaret Lee Runbeck

"You can lead a horse to the water, but you can't make it drink." – Unknown

"Pain is inevitable. Misery is optional." – Hyrum W. Smith

"I do not take a single newspaper, nor read one a month, and I feel myself infinitely the happier for it. The man who reads nothing at all is better educated than the man who reads nothing but newspapers." – Thomas Jefferson

"One of the first duties of the physician is to educate the masses not to take medicine." – Sir William Osler

"Few people are logical. Most of us are prejudiced and biased... Most people don't want to change their minds. We are not creatures of logic we are creatures of emotions." – Dale Carnegie

Personal Thank Yous

First and above all, I would like to thank my Lord and Savior Jesus Christ. Without God, none of this would be possible. Thank you, God, for blessing me with the power to control and direct my own mind to whatever I desire.

I would like to thank my parents, George E. Booker and Clara L. Booker, for bringing me into this world. I understand you two planned my birth and wanted me to be born on May 19, my dad's birthday. Sorry I was born two days late on May 21. ☺ Thanks for all your support and everything you two have done for me. I love you both, Mom and Dad.

To my sisters, Donna J. Adams, Michelle D. Booker, and Judith L. Evans, and my brother, Clarence E. Booker. Thank you guys for everything. Your thoughts and words about me are extremely motivational. I don't think I would have made it this far without you guys!! Keep spreading the word about me! I love you all!!

To my late grandmother, Geraldine B. Heard, who indirectly taught me the importance of kindness and forgiveness, and directly told me to never give up. Thanks, Granny. I love you so much!

To the Dillard family, especially the late Thelma Dillard, who often called me "Our other child" and would always say, "Never make yourself common." And to Valerie Dillard for always

treating me like a son. Thanks
for your kindness and
generosity. I learned a lot of
family values from the Dillards.
I love you all!

To the late, great Mrs. Earline
Brooks, who I wish was still with
us so she could see me now. Mrs.
Brooks was always about
uplifting her community and
the children in it. She saw
potential in me when not many
others did. Mrs. Brooks formed a
neighborhood street watch for
adults and also a Jr. street club
for the next generation and
made me president of that Jr.
club. She always told me I would
be someone special. We met once

a week in her home and talked about so many things. She fed us, gave us snacks, juice, and even money. She even took us multiple places at her expense. And one of the most fascinating experiences we had was Christmas caroling! Walking up and down the street singing Christmas songs with lit candles was a wonderful experience. Thank you so much for everything you instilled in us. I love you!

To the late Mama Sally, who also treated us very special with the peanut butter cookies she would bake on a regular basis. Thank you so much for your kindness. I love you!

Another very special thank you to the late Mrs. Thompson and her sweet daughter Sylvinia Thompson, a.k.a. Nana, who would always give me treats and take me sled riding and skiing. These sweet women also taught me how to plant and grow my own garden. To this day, I still love to grow my own fruits, vegetables, and herbs. Thank you so very much. I love you all!

Special thanks to my church home, St. Agnes Our Lady of Fatima, and my wonderful pastor and friend Rev. Robert Marva. Thank you so much for being a mentor to me and helping me through so many difficult times. Your encouraging words of wisdom have lifted my spirits many times when I was ready to give up. Thanks, Father Bob! I love you!

To Antoinette Smith, who refuses to allow me to feel bad in any situation and always offers the perfect words and smile to remind me that all is well. Thank you very much. I love you!

This is a very unusual thank you, but it must be done. My second week in prison, I beat this dude up pretty bad. I was unaware of some of the "prison rules," and Antoine Winn, a.k.a. Fess, who was asleep at the time of the fight, saved my life. Fess overheard a group of guys planning on shanking me up. For all who don't know what that means, it's stabbing me, in so many words. He told those dudes I was untouchable, and they would have to go through him in order to get to me! After his conversation with them, he came to me and explained I wasn't on the streets and prison life is a lot different. Being the hot head I was, I flared up at him, and before I could utter any words, he grabbed me by the throat and said, "Man these niggas plotting on killing your lil wild ass, and I just put my life on the line for you." My heart dropped, and I felt a fear I had never felt in my life. After he and I talked, he walked me up to those dudes to squash the beef. He also spent the rest of that day introducing me to everyone he felt I may have a problem with. I would probably be dead if it wasn't for him. Thanks, Fess! That was a real Wade Park OG call. Much love!

To the late Stephanie Collins, who always believed in me and would always tell me I was special and would grow up to be somebody special. She also always used to have these short conversations with me that I refuse to reveal. Thank you so much. You are truly missed. I love you!

To my auntie Helen Wilson, a.k.a. Marcie, thanks for the valuable weekends I spent with you and the money you would pay me for washing dishes and going grocery shopping with you. I love you!

To my BIG CUZ Terran Wilson, "TANK," thanks for not beating me up for stealing cassettes and cologne. LOL; honestly, I didn't know any better.

To Mike Trivisonno, Eric
Smedley, Viola Jackson, Donna
Blythewood, Irwin "Swirv"
Dillard, DoRhonda Unichi,
Terry Sigler, Corlette Rudolph,
James Evans Sr., Sandra Gay,
Yvonne Williamson, Maurice
Dancie, Luther Manghum,
Maurice Craddock, Mr. Reed,
Deborah James and the James
family, Elinor Williamson,
Tonya Owens, Maria Welborne,
Chris Austin, the late Ralph
Shaft, Irvin Bostic, Lashone
Stewart, my late cousin Bobbette
Heard, my sweet cousin Barbara
Carter, my nieces and nephews,
my uncles the late Charles
Heard, Lawrence Heard, Joseph
Heard, Phillip Heard, and my

aunties Ann Marie Heard, Marilyn Robertson, and Barbara Heard, thank you all for your support and kind words. Thank you all for never judging me and listening to bullshit gossip. Thank you all for believing in me. I love you all.

To all my cousins and the rest of my family and true friends who I failed to mention, I thank you as well. I sincerely love you all!

Can't forget about these people:

To everyone who told me as a child I wouldn't amount to anything; to all who gossiped

about me, spreading false
rumors; to the people who taught
me to steal from others and who
stole from me; the teachers,
counselors, principals,
administrators, and other staff
members who also said I
wouldn't amount to anything or
would be dead or in jail before
twenty-one; all the corrections
officers who told me I would be
back in prison; the EPD for
framing me and falsifying police
reports; and the Cleveland police
officers who shot at me while I
was running away unarmed; all
my haters; the mothers of my
children who ruined a father and
child relationship; all you fake-
ass friends who talk behind my
back then smile in my face, and

all the fake-ass friends who stole CDs, guns, drugs, pictures, and money from me, especially the ones who stole out of my car when I gave you rides; and last but not least, everyone who told me no when I needed a yes—to each and every one of y'all:

I salute the Divinity in you!

About The Author

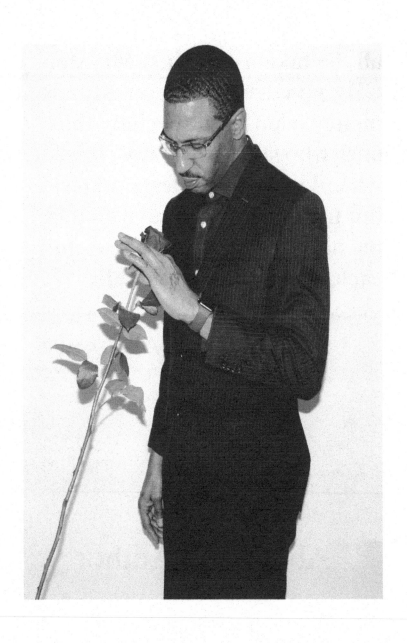

George E. Booker II is widely regarded as one of the world's leading researchers in the field of health care and many other controversial topics. He is rapidly becoming the nation's premier consumer advocate and exposer of corporate corruption. George is actively pursuing foundations and individuals to help fight against these corrupt corporations and government agencies. Mr. Booker currently resides in Euclid, Ohio.

Death comes to us all. At some point in each of our lives, we must experience death, not knowing how or when. A friend or family member must depart from us. One day, it will be you! Well, unfortunately, on 06-02-2016, several innocent people were injured and my big brother Clarence Edward Booker departed in a tragic six-car accident, which may have been caused by a drunk driver. Please don't think I'm pointing the finger at the impaired driver. I'm not blaming her at all. I want you all to understand the impact on other people lives

when someone drinks alcohol
and drives a car. DON'T
DRINK AND DRIVE! Please
act more responsibly, people.
Your actions may result in
someone's death.
DON'T DRINK AND DRIVE!

RIP
Clarence E. Booker

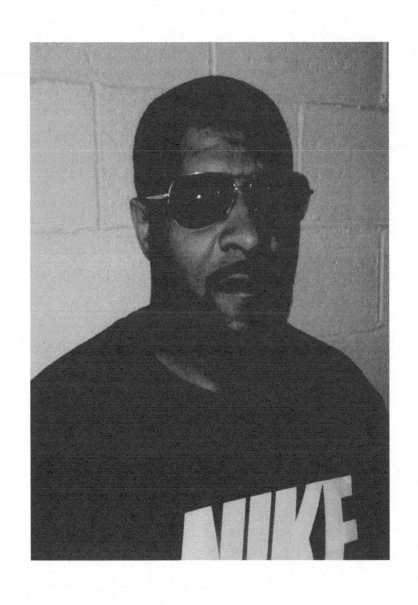

I Love You, Big Bro!